T0147088

KINGDOM
Fitness

KEVIN MCCRARY

WESTBOW
P R E S S°
A DIVISION OF THOMAS NELSON
& ZONDERVAN

Copyright © 2022 Kevin McCrary.

All rights reserved. No part of this book may be used or reproduced by any means, graphic, electronic, or mechanical, including photocopying, recording, taping or by any information storage retrieval system without the written permission of the author except in the case of brief quotations embodied in critical articles and reviews.

This book is a work of non-fiction. Unless otherwise noted, the author and the publisher make no explicit guarantees as to the accuracy of the information contained in this book and in some cases, names of people and places have been altered to protect their privacy.

WestBow Press books may be ordered through booksellers or by contacting:

WestBow Press
A Division of Thomas Nelson & Zondervan
1663 Liberty Drive
Bloomington, IN 47403
www.westbowpress.com
844-714-3454

Because of the dynamic nature of the Internet, any web addresses or links contained in this book may have changed since publication and may no longer be valid. The views expressed in this work are solely those of the author and do not necessarily reflect the views of the publisher, and the publisher hereby disclaims any responsibility for them.

Any people depicted in stock imagery provided by Getty Images are models, and such images are being used for illustrative purposes only. Certain stock imagery © Getty Images.

Scripture marked (KJV) taken from the King James Version of the Bible.

Scripture quotations marked (NIV) are taken from the Holy Bible, New International Version®, NIV®. Copyright © 1973, 1978, 1984, 2011 by Biblica, Inc.® Used by permission of Zondervan. All rights reserved worldwide. www.zondervan.com The "NIV" and "New International Version" are trademarks registered in the United States Patent and Trademark Office by Biblica, Inc.®

Scripture marked by (NKJV) taken from the New King James Version®. Copyright © 1982 by Thomas Nelson. Used by permission. All rights reserved.

ISBN: 978-1-6642-4784-0 (sc)
ISBN: 978-1-6642-4786-4 (hc)
ISBN: 978-1-6642-4785-7 (e)

Library of Congress Control Number: 2021921442

Print information available on the last page.

WestBow Press rev. date: 07/28/2022

Thank you, Lord, for this revelation. I pray that this word fulfills the assignment you have called it to in the hearts and lives of your people.

Amen.

CONTENTS

PREFACE
KINGDOM FITNESS

The diet and weight loss industry is a multibillion dollar a year business and continues to grow, yet there is still a consistent rise in obesity and the overall unhealthiness of our society. The United States of America is rated as one of the most obese countries in the world, and in some studies it's the most obese nation at over 36% according to 2020 data from the OECD (Organization for Economic Cooperation and Development). Some studies differ, but the point is we are always in the discussion, despite our obsession with health and fitness. This is an alarming statistic that can be witnessed in members of our society as early as childhood. We have grown up in a society that puts a tremendous amount of pressure upon us to produce a certain image— to convince us to buy into their miracle pills, specialized diets, faulty workout programs, unnecessary medical procedures, and more.

Western culture bases health and fitness around convenience, appearance, and quick results—so much so that we allow it to dictate, along with people's opinions of us, who we are or can be. When the truth about an issue is revealed, only then can it be truly addressed. Until then it is understandable, to a degree, why our society is in the state it is.

My people are destroyed for lack of knowledge: because thou hast rejected knowledge, I will also reject thee, that thou shalt be no priest to me: seeing that thou has forgotten the law of thy God, I will also forget thy children. (Hosea 4:6 KJV)

This scripture stands true now concerning every area of our lives in which we reject knowledge. The knowledge I'm referring to is that of God. Everything we see in the natural realm has been established by God first in the spiritual realm. We can't have truth without Him; therefore, we can't establish a standard by which to live without Him. Humanity has rejected God and His word, so He has rejected us. Now we suffer because of it. That doesn't mean He lacks love for or is out to punish us, but rather He will not force himself upon us when we reject Him. We must open ourselves up to the truth of God.

Take a few moments right now, and envision your dream car. What if you spend long, hard hours working toward purchasing that vehicle? You take any overtime hours available and save every penny you can spare. Over the course of the next several years you make sure your credit is in good standing, and you do all you possibly can to be able to purchase it. The day finally comes when you can get what you've worked so hard for. You make your way down to the dealership, and with great anticipation and satisfaction, you buy the car of your dreams.

After you sign on the dotted line, you hop into your dream car and put the keys in the ignition, but as soon as you turn the ignition switch the car spits you out and tells you with confidence and in full rebellion that it is not a car and refuses to be driven. Sounds ridiculous, right? But we do just the same when we try to establish our lives without the truth of God.

Health is no exception to this rule! Everything about your dream car—its frame, the way it functions, its color, the dos and don'ts—are all dictated by the manufacturer, or simply, *the Creator*. If you put sweet tea in the gas tank it wouldn't fuel your car to move, let alone start. If you put anything into the vehicle that shouldn't be there, it would fail to produce. Why? The vehicle was not set by those standards or for any other purpose.

In continuing outside of the set standards, you'll limit what it could do for you. It still has all the features and qualities as advertised, but because it is not being taken care of properly and is not being used according to the manufacturer's set standard, it will not fulfill its created purpose.

My assignment is to bring to light that we were created by God for His purposes and not by man. There is a design from God concerning our health. He was not aimless in His creation of us, nor were we created out of spontaneous and random acts of nature. If viewed correctly, this truth causes us to take our hope out of man's limited hands and seek a higher authority on the matter. With that said, there's no higher authority than that which we find in God and His holy scripture. I petition you today to consider trusting in the only one who can truly address this matter.

My assignment is to cause a paradigm shift in the way you view health and fitness. This kingdom mindset, if applied correctly, will cause you to live a healthier and more fruitful life not dependent on worldly means. This is not a book about diets or a militant exercise craze. This is about empowering people to pursue better, healthier lives full of purpose and potential. Welcome to *Kingdom Fitness*!

ACKNOWLEDGMENTS

For God so loved the world that he gave his only begotten Son, that
whosoever believeth in him shall not perish, but have everlasting life.
—John 3:16 (KJV)

Thank you, Jesus, for the finished work of the cross and for your evident
love and hand in my life.

To my parents, Thomas and Hannah McCrary, for all the sacrifices you have
made and the example you've set for your children. I love and thank you!

To my siblings Lavert, Eldon, Lambert, Tammie, Deborah, and Tonja
and to all my family and friends—I love you very much, and I appreciate
the parts each of you have played in my life!

To Bishop RJ Matthews and my church family Kingdom Vision,
thank you for all you have poured into me. The amount of growth I've
experienced in Christ since I've been connected to this body is priceless.

To my daughter, Norah—you are so precious in my sight. I love you and
pray that this book be a reminder to you of the strength God has given
you to be a mighty deliverer and standard in your generation.

To my wife, Cindy—you are the love of my life. You are my best friend
and my biggest supporter. I love you and want you to know that I am
with you as you pursue all God has called you to be and do!

INTRODUCTION
CHANGE YOUR MIND

From that time Jesus began to preach, and to say,
repent: For the Kingdom of Heaven is at hand.
—Matthew 4:17 (KJV)

This scripture is in reference to the kingdom of God. We are going to focus on the word *repent*. To repent means to turn away from sin, rebelliousness, or disobedience and turn instead to God. It means to have a change of mind from the way we think and do things to God's way. The kingdom of God adheres to His standard and His government.

In this scripture Jesus confronted people with a command to repent. This expresses that, in order to receive what God has for them, for people to truly live, their minds must change. You must change the way you think, live, and do things. This will require a sincere repentance of the heart and mind, which in the culture of that day were one in the same. The command to repent (change your mind) is required of us all in every area of our lives, especially the areas where we wish to see the fruits of God's kingdom expressed the most. Whenever something from the kingdom of God is introduced, it takes letting go of what we think we know in order to grab hold of what is presented to us. We have done things the world's way long enough; it's time for a change!

Fitness is about being physically fit to fulfill that which one has been put on this earth by God to do. By using God's standard there is a state of health. In both the spiritual and the natural we have access to what we need to take our lives to the next level. In order to do that we must change our minds, the way we think, and what we have been taught, submitting ourselves totally to the government of God.

In the world today, the demand for quick fixes leads the way in motivating us to set unrealistic goals to enhance our health. We depend largely on the knowledge of humans and their governments, which are absent from God's revelations and answers. We expect them to tell the truth and look out for our best interests, but we have placed our trust in the hands of the fallen, who have rejected the knowledge of God. With that said, there could be a number of factors that have facilitated our current condition. We can point fingers at what or who we feel is to blame—and might have valid arguments to a degree—but when it comes down to the core of the problem, it's us.

It's our responsibility to be intentional about our own health and at least fact-check what is presented to us as truth. The answers to our problems as they pertain to health often hinge around what we are or are not doing. What we do or don't know has led us to where we are. So many people have settled and given themselves over to lies and incomplete information—some to the point of giving up or even losing their lives. That withstanding, no matter your condition, disappointment, or discouraging experience, whether it's mental, physical, or spiritual, there is hope!

One
INTELLIGENT DESIGN

Whether one believes in God or not, I think it's safe to say we didn't evolve from apes nor did a big explosion of organisms form us, as some theories suggest. At least it didn't happen in the way they think. I don't care how you do the math—nothing always produces nothing. Nothingness has no ability within itself to produce anything other than what it already is. Nothing! Only when an extant force introduces something new does change occur in said equation. In other words, you can add, subtract, multiply, or divide nothing into nothing, and the only result would be nothing. If a door is shut, it will remain that way until another factor has been added to that equation to cause it to open.

I don't know about you, but an explosive force (big bang theory) or a sudden appearance sounds an awful lot like what will happen if an extant force (God) speaks to an equation of zero and changes it from nothing to something. Have you ever taken a serious look at our bodies and how truly complex they are? Consider the fact that we have not discovered everything there is to know about them and how they function. It should be evident to us that there is more to our being than the world teaches us.

> "So God created man in His own image, in the image of God created He him; male and female created He them" (Genesis 1:27 KJV).

This scripture begs the question that if God created us, why are we using human solutions to fix a God-made body? We have made a habit of rejecting what we don't understand or can't control. We are desperate for answers and are quick to accept what is presented to us as the truth. Our minds have developed in many ways to fill in the blanks when truth is not known or we're asked to comprehend an experience that challenges it. Instead of seeking to understand an issue, we try to put it into a neat box that keeps it from changing our little world.

We adopt ideals that conveniently fit our situation, good or bad. We often accept things we shouldn't as the gospel truth because it's easier to believe due to our limited experience. As we proceed further, my prayer is that the Lord will open your heart and eyes and increase your faith so that you can receive what He has for you.

One of the biggest problems people have with believing we are creations of God is that it forces us out of a lot of excuses. A belief in a higher authority confronts complacency and trust in oneself. It causes us to live to a higher standard and be held accountable for our own actions. It gives boundaries, purpose, and order to our lives. Without those boundaries and that order, we live recklessly and misuse the freedom we have. Without purpose, we wander aimlessly. "Sometimes the greatest bondage can be freedom," said Bishop RJ Matthews. Show me a society without purpose, order, and boundaries, and I will show a place headed for destruction.

It's the same outcome when there are disorders in our bodies. If we want to get to the core of what state our bodies best function in, we must go to the Creator, our Maker. What does He have to say about the issue? We must ask ourselves, *Do we believe in God, and do we trust what He teaches us in His word*? This doesn't mean we disregard the counsel of those, like doctors, who have been given the wisdom by God to understand the body, but we are not to depend on them solely. The greatest responsibility for our well-being belongs to us, and we must depend on the Creator to instruct us on properly keeping it. We must come to the understanding that to live a healthy life full of purpose, we must go to the one who has given us life and a purpose and grab hold of—not only the spiritual things—but also what He has given us to practically apply to our everyday lives. If we accept this truth, we are on our way to finding the solution to our personal health issues.

In the first two chapters of Genesis, the Bible explains the process of creation and how God was well pleased with everything He had created. Genesis 3 begins to discuss the fall of man. Before the fall, everything God created was perfect, just as He intended it. This included the first man, Adam, and the first woman, Eve. Everything about them—the way they lived, their walk, and their health—was in perfect alignment with the will of God. They had uninterrupted communion with God and all they needed to continue in the same way. It was not until the fall of man—the entering of sin—that all of this changed. Because sin was introduced when God's boundaries were disregarded in the garden, they found themselves separated from Him. They sinned against God and found themselves separated from their true source of life, which caused them to be susceptible to immorality, sickness, and death. As the first man and woman, they set in motion generations ago what we experience today.

In Genesis 3, there is a powerful revelation about the effects of humankind being separated from the Lord. In verses 9–10 of chapter 3, God calls for Adam after he and Eve disobeyed God's command about the tree whose fruit they were forbidden to eat (the boundary that was set) in the garden. Adam's response was very interesting to me. Adam responded, "I heard your voice in the garden, and I was afraid, because I was naked" (Genesis 3:10 NIV). Let's highlight the word *naked,* considering that is what Adam was before his disobedience—naked! So what changed that made this time different?

Before they disobeyed God, they had no fear or shame. They operated with dominion and purpose. They did not operate in insecurity, nor were they unable to fulfill what God had called them to do. The understanding after they sinned that they were naked was not a picture of their obvious physical state. They were naked the whole time without it being an issue. Instead, it was a revelation concerning their now fallen state.

The Oxford English Dictionary describes *naked* as being without usual covering or protection, being devoid of, exposed to harm, or being vulnerable. *Merriam Webster's Collegiate Dictionary* describes it as being scantily supplied or furnished, lacking embellishment, unarmed, defenseless, or not being backed by the writer's ownership of the commodity contract or security. In other words, what was being expressed by Adam through his response to God was what was going on in him spiritually as a result of being separated from God. This is important because when God leaves, or if there is separation from Him, so does every benefit of having a relationship with Him. We are suddenly unequipped to be or to do what He has created us to. *Merriam Webster's Collegiate Dictionary* also gives one of the synonyms for the word *naked* as *being barren,* which means being incapable of producing offspring; habitually failing to fruit; desolate; lacking inspiration or ideas; devoid; lacking interest or charm.

At this point, Adam was so insecure and so far from who he was created to be that two verses later (Genesis 3:1–12 NIV), he blames God and throws his wife, Eve, under the bus for his actions. Where we are separated from God in life, we become unequipped to properly deal with problems or challenges in that area. Just think of God as the earth and us as a strong tree rooted deeply in Him. If we are rooted in the earth, we can produce fruit and seed for more trees and fruit. We can withstand the heat of the summer and cold of the winter, adapting to every season while enduring the different storms that are produced in our environment. We can provide shade and shelter for people and wildlife, but if you were to uproot us and place us on a slab of concrete in a store parking lot, we would suddenly be unequipped for life and would eventually get sick and die. It wouldn't matter how much you watered us or how much we danced, sang, and prayed; if we are not rooted in the earth (God), we would eventually get sick and die.

In taking a closer examination of scripture and looking from that time until now, there is an ongoing trend that gets worse with every generation. From the time of humans' first transgression, we begin to see more and more immoral behavior, sicknesses sprouting up, and the life span of humans beginning to decrease. With all of that said, there is hope! Why am I so optimistic about there being hope? There is no such thing as a problem without a solution in the kingdom of God. For there to be a problem, there has to be a previous state of right standing! If not so, then where lies the problem?

> "For God so loved the world, that He gave His only begotten Son, that whosoever believeth in Him should not perish, but have everlasting life" (John 3:16 KJV).

By receiving Christ Jesus as our Lord and Savior, we have now been reconciled unto God, and the separation from Him that once was has now been bridged through Jesus. If one is willing, this allows God to work not only supernaturally but also practically in our lives, giving us access to healing through the revelation of who He is. Jesus puts us in a position of right standing with God that makes all things possible to those who believe in His name.

It is very interesting to me that no matter how many medical advances our society makes it's not enough to stop the increase in early deaths due to unhealthy lifestyles.

> Let no man deceive himself. If any man among you seemeth to be wise in this world, let him become a fool, that he may be wise. For the wisdom of this world is foolishness with God. For it is written, He taketh the wise in their own craftiness. And again, The Lord knoweth the thoughts of the wise, that they are vain. Therefore let no man glory in men. For all things are yours; Whether Paul, or Aplollos, or cephas, or the world, or life, or death, or things present, or things to come; all are yours; and ye are Christ's; and Christ is God's. (1 Corinthians 3:18–23 KJV)

Anything that does not have Christ as its foundation will leave you with false or incomplete information leading ultimately to death in that area.

> "For other foundation can no man lay than that is laid, which is Jesus Christ" (1 Corinthians 3:11 KJV).

When you look at your current state of health, can you say it was built on a solid foundation? Or has it been built upon what society has taught you? If the world really knew, would we be in our current state?

Two

PERISHING

From the time of our separation from God through sin, there has been a constant rise in people leaving before their appointed time. Fathers, mothers, sons, and daughters alike are leaving us. This no doubt has affected many lives in a negative way. We know that it is appointed for all once to die (Hebrews 9:27) and that it is a part of life, but there are a great number of deaths occurring on account of our free will. A great deal of it has to do with a lack of knowledge concerning a healthy lifestyle. This not only affects the quality of our lives, but also those lives God has called us to touch.

Without proper knowledge we perish and, sadly, many do so with unfinished business, like leaving loved ones behind in a bad financial situation or leaving a child without one or both of their parents. In many cases parents have had to bury their own children. The list is endless when observing the consequences of a devastating illness or untimely death.

Hosea 4:6 (KJV) says, "My people are destroyed for the lack of knowledge." That is the awareness of facts, truths, or principles set in motion by God at the beginning of what mankind knows as existence. There are facts and principles we should live by in order to attain and maintain a healthy body. There are undeniable truths that we must apply. Being ignorant of those truths does not give us a free pass to live however we want. It is our responsibility to seek knowledge for our lives.

"The heart of him that hath understanding seeketh knowledge" (Proverbs 15:14 KJV).

"A wise man is strong: yea, a man of knowledge increaseth strength" (Proverbs 24:5 KJV).

All of us need to take the time to invest in knowledge that will improve our health. Knowledge applied to our lives concerning health will increase productivity and the overall enjoyment we experience.

Most of us have heard the expression "Knowledge is power." That power in and of itself is of no benefit to me unless I tap into it. I can only benefit from the knowledge I'm willing to apply. "For faith without works (application) is dead" (James 2:20 KJV). When we don't apply knowledge, we're bound by our current state of living and or thinking.

"The Excellency of knowledge is that wisdom giveth life to them that have it" (Ecclesiastes 7:12 KJV).

"Every prudent (wise) man deals with knowledge" (Proverbs 13:16 KJV).

I encourage you to not just get knowledge but to apply it as well. You will be blessed by the benefits, and more importantly, others will be blessed by what God has put inside you for their benefit.

Everything we build in this life should be done with a proper reverence for God. We should be able to measure the truth of a matter by the standard of God.

This is both a spiritual and physical principle. When we are separated from God in any area of our life, sickness, disease and eventually death will creep in.

Jesus stated, "I have come that they may have life, and that they may have it more abundantly" (John 10:10 NKJV). A plenteous life! It is in receiving and following Jesus that we find this abundant life. As already stated in this book, when you need something fixed that has been broken you go to the manufacturer of that product, the creator of it, to fix it. So must we go to our Creator to know what is beneficial for us and what is not. In Him we will truly learn how to take care of and benefit from the body with which He has blessed us!

As I've applied this truth to my life, I have found that many areas in the field of health are faulty based on their foundation leading to more problems down the line. There is only one road to the truth, and that is through Christ Jesus. Building our lives on anything other than God and His word is faulty and will crumble under the pressures of life. Why should we trust God and His word above man's wisdom void of God?

> "In the beginning was the Word, and the Word was with God, and the Word was God. He was with God in the beginning. Through Him all things were made; without Him nothing was made that has been made" (John 1:1–3 NIV).

> "All people are like grass, and all their glory is like the flowers of the field; the grass withers and the flowers fall, but the word of the Lord endures forever." (1 Peter 1:24–25 NIV)

> "Heaven and earth shall pass away, but my words shall not pass away" (Matthew 24:35 KJV).

"Man shall not live by bread alone, but by every word that proceeds out of the mouth of God" (Matthew 4:4 KJV).

Everything we build as believers should be measured by and built on the foundation that is Christ Jesus! Ephesians 2:20 refers to Jesus as the "chief cornerstone," also known as the foundation stone. Any building built on anything other than a strong foundation will eventually collapse due to the weight of the building itself or from its surrounding environment.

The lack of a strong foundation leads to an inability to manage, making one vulnerable to giving up or giving in to dangerous ideologies. We can't expect the world to care about the things of God and because they do not care for the things of Him, they will not carry His heart, His standard nor the truth of His word on an issue. But what if they have noble intentions? "All of us have become like one who is unclean, and all our righteous acts are like filthy rags; we all shrivel up like a leaf, and like the wind our sins sweep us away" (Isaiah 64:6 NIV).

> Those who live according to the flesh have their minds set on what the flesh desires; but those who live in accordance with the Spirit have their minds set on what the Spirit desires. The mind governed by the flesh is death, but the mind governed by the Spirit is life and peace. The mind governed by the flesh is hostile to God; it does not submit to God's law, nor can it do so. Those who are in the realm of the flesh cannot please God. (Romans 8:7–8 NIV)

If a man is unrighteous his actions will follow suit in the corruption of the truth. This is not to say that every person who doesn't believe as we do is after us or has no knowledge. But we as believers cannot build our life by the direction of people who deny Jesus. Our very lives were put together by kingdom principles. These are spiritual principles of God that affect everything around us.

We must measure what is told to us as truth against the standard of God, because Satan is the master of deception. He cannot create, so instead he makes a copy of the truth. He creates a version so close to the truth that if you don't do your homework, he will convince you of it.

We must remind ourselves that our lives ultimately are not about us. There are souls attached to the purpose God has put inside us. The world needs what God has placed on the inside of you; therefore, getting knowledge and using it correctly is your responsibility and of great importance.

> Do you not know that your bodies are temples of the Holy Spirit, who is in you, whom you have received from God? You are not your own; you were bought at a price. Therefore, honor God with your bodies. (1 Corinthians 6:19–20 NIV)

When we accept Jesus as our Lord and Savior, His spirit comes to live inside us; therefore, we must operate as good stewards of what He has given us. The majority of all Christians know this (or should), but few truly adhere to it. When we know what God has said and don't respond rightly, we are in rebellion. Rebellion is one having a resisting spirit to authority. "Rebellion is a key principle of Satan!" (Bishop R. J. Matthews). In scripture, rebellion is described as the sin of witchcraft (1 Samuel 15:23).

Ignorance, when we can seek out and attain knowledge, is not an excuse beyond childhood. When we're children, we must be trained in the way to go, but as we get older, we must apply discipline to our lives, for our responsibilities are greater.

Many of the issues we deal with in our bodies don't just happen upon us. Our lifestyles facilitated them. Because these habits are started earlier with each generation, the manifestations are greater and more frequent. When a child is conceived, it draws from what the mother and father have provided through genetics, and those genes are affected by the ones before them and what their lifestyles were as well—good or bad.

While a child is being carried by its mother, it lives off the nourishment the mother provides. When the child is born it still does not decide on what's consumed. Parents play a larger role in the development of their children's health than they think. Granted, we can't control everything, and there are other factors like stress and pollution that may affect the health of our offspring. But we can still make positive changes to help.

Please do not come unto condemnation. It's impossible for someone to control what's been done throughout generations of their family line that affects those after. Just do your part in getting things back on track.

When I was a child my mother fed me and my siblings plenty of fruits and vegetables. They did not always taste as good to me as other food options nor did they always look as appealing. Over a course of time I developed a palate for them because my mother continued to feed us that way. She was brought up that way as a child and ate that way while she was pregnant with me. As I grew, I continued in that way.

> "Train up a child in the way that he should go and when he is old he shall not depart from it" (Proverbs 22:6 KJV).

My mom got applied knowledge from her parents, and then she applied and passed it on to my brothers, my sister, and I, who are actively passing it on to the next generation. Even though we have not been perfect in this, the habits and knowledge are being reproduced in the next generation. Remember that when you choose to not get knowledge and apply it; it affects more than just you and possibly even many generations into the future.

It may not be easy, and you may find yourself angry because the ones before you didn't know, but now as you learn the truth, you can make a positive change. You may be the one who has to do all the groundwork building the foundation for it. Just know that what you do is going to echo throughout the generations to come. The beauty of it is that with each generation the knowledge is greater and becomes easier to apply. Know that God is with you and wants you to be healthy so you can live a healthy and purposeful life.

> "Grace and peace be yours in abundance through the knowledge of God and of Jesus our Lord. His divine power has given us everything we need for a godly life through our knowledge of Him who called us by His own glory and goodness" (2 Peter 1:2–3 NIV).

> "I can do all things through Christ who strengthens me" (Philippians 4:1 NKJV).

Three

FALSE PROPHETS

Beloved, believe not every spirit, but try the spirits whether they are of God: because many false prophets are gone out into the world.
—1 John 4:1 (KJV)

For the time will come when people will not put up with sound doctrine. Instead, to suit their own desires, they will gather around them a great number of teachers to say what their itching ears want to hear. They will turn their ears away from the truth and turn aside to myths.
—2 Timothy 4:3–4 (NIV)

A prophet is a spokesman for God who communicates His messages to chosen people. A false prophet on the other hand looks to deceive and manipulate through what may not always seem like an evident lie. They pervert the truth by twisting it to fit their own personal agenda taking advantage of the vulnerable. Anyone who is marketing something to be the truth when it is not should be considered a false prophet. Anything presented that is in opposition to God or his holy word is false.

Hereby know ye the Spirit of God: Every spirit that confesseth that Jesus Christ is come in the flesh is of God: And every spirit that confesseth not that Jesus Christ is come in the flesh is not of God: and this is the spirit of antichrist, whereof ye have heard that it should come; and even now already is it in the world. (1 John 4:2-3 KJV)

Remember God has established everything by divine principles by which we are to govern ourselves. These principles cannot be reversed or changed by man. The validity of what we are being presented should be checked against the word of God. Any form of doctrine being taught that is contrary to the word of God is false. This doesn't always mean someone intends to mislead, but when you separate life issues from the One who created life you're actively taking the truth out of the equation, which hinders your ability to properly address a situation. True health is in God through Christ Jesus working in us.

We must remember that whatever is not of God will never draw us to dependency on Him but only separate us from Him, allowing sickness and death to come into our lives. He is our life source. Just as the roots of a tree need the earth, so we need God.

How can I speak this in boldness? The truth is all around us. Despite all the technological, scientific, and medical advances humans have made, all the different exercise routines and diet plans we have, we are a world that consistently sees health issues arise in it. In our own wisdom, void of God, we have been under the false impression that we have really been achieving something when we have done nothing more than put a Band-Aid on a bullet wound.

We have cheated ourselves and those whose needs we were created to meet because we refuse to seek God on these matters, and we've allowed people who don't have His will at heart to convince us their ways are better. There is only one love—that which we receive in Christ Jesus. Anyone void of Him cannot produce that type of love nor the revelation that comes through that relationship. Therefore, they do not have the capability of producing a complete truth, which should be our standard.

For His word declares we are complete in Him (Colossians 2:10). God is the Creator, and without the Creator we can't truly create! Neither can the world and its prophets create, let alone complete!

We must beware of every idea or belief presented to us by these false prophets. They present to us help under the pretense of innocence and concern but underneath in the spiritual the enemy is at work trying to cause our demise (Matthew 7:15). We must remind ourselves that no matter someone's good intentions, if they are void of a relationship dependent on God, it is impossible for them to produce the things of God. This is not an attack on people but on the spirits behind the people and their motives.

> For we wrestle not against flesh and blood, but against principalities, against powers, against the rulers of the darkness of this world, against spiritual wickedness in high places. (Ephesians 6:12 KJV)

The bible teaches us to stand having our loins girded about with truth (Ephesians 6:14). This scripture is in reference to a leather belt that military soldiers in that time wore that held in place and supported most of the pieces of their armor. The revelation that we receive from God will hold everything together. What is of the truth shall stand. "For false Christs and false prophets shall rise, and shall shew signs and wonders, to seduce, if it were possible even the elect" (Mark 13:22 KJV).

Diets, diet pills, and different procedures that are not natural for the body to undergo should be avoided.

> But there were false prophets also among the people, even as there shall be false teachers among you, who privily shall bring in damnable heresies, even denying

the Lord that bought them, and bring upon themselves swift destruction. (2 Peter 2:1 KJV)

In our school systems they teach the theory of evolution to our kids, along with other false doctrines and ideals while at the same time pushing out God and prayer. "Many shall follow their pernicious ways; by reason of whom the way of truth shall be evil spoken of" (2 Peter 2:2 KJV).

We are seeing more and more dishonor and hatred for God and His ways.

We cannot give into it! We must not leave our lives in the hands of those who can't give life. Our lives and the purpose placed in us are gifts from God and are of great value to Him. He loves us and wants what's best for us. We must be cautious concerning what we allow ourselves to receive as the truth. We must look at the fruit, whether it is of God or not, for the word declares that we shall know them (false prophets) by their fruit (Matthew 7:20). So "beware lest any man spoil you through philosophy and vain deceit, after the tradition of men, after the rudiments of the world and not after Christ" (Colossians 2:8 KJV).

Four

CREATED FOR PURPOSE

If you're like me in any way, you probably require a reason for most of the things you invest time, money and effort into. You need a reason why! Why workout? Why take care of my body and change my eating habits? Of what value is it to my life? Even as a physically active person I still find the need to have a reason to eat right and take care of my body in order to maintain consistent motivation toward a healthy lifestyle. I'm a personal fitness trainer; I served in the US Army, and I participate in plenty of sports—basketball more than any, yet I still need a reason. I need a purpose!

God created the earth and everything in it with a purpose in mind. A purpose is something set up with a desired end to be attained. It's a resolution, an intention, and a determination. A purpose is an object or result aimed at or achieved. It's reason for doing something. A purpose can drive our life to a place we've never been before, giving us vitality, hope, and a meaning in life. Having no purpose—or worse, not realizing we have one—greatly affects our lives. Not having a purpose causes us to make bad relationship choices. Not having a sense of purpose can cause us to devalue education or responsibility. Having a sense of purpose can be the difference between someone robbing you and instead providing a service to you. It is the difference between a child who grew up in a bad environment taking another's life out of frustration and instead saving a life because now he or she is a doctor.

The thief cometh not, but for to steal, and to kill, and to destroy: I am come that they might have life, and that they might have it more abundantly. (John 10:10 KJV)

Christ has come to give us an abundant life and purpose—a meaning we won't find from any other person, place, or thing. We should ask God several times throughout our lives, such as, *Who are You? Who am I in You? What have You put me here to do?* When we get a revelation of that we will find purpose. God has a plan for our lives individually that is part of what He desires to bring forth collectively through His people. "And we know that all things work together for good to them that love God, to them who are the called according to His purpose" Romans 8:28 (KJV).

Having a toned body with six-pack abs looks great, but if that's all you have to offer me, it's not good enough. It's not meaningful enough to sustain me because its basis is vanity. That won't make me get up and work out when I don't feel like it. It won't make me fit a session into a tight schedule.

Until we are able to find a purpose that drives us, we will find it hard to do what we need consistently enough to get physically fit and stay there. Purpose puts into perspective that it's a lifestyle change and not just a phase or event we participate in occasionally. This is important because what you don't take care of the enemy will take advantage of!

When I was in the military I attended a revival service at a local church just outside of my duty station. The keynote speaker at the end of his message posed a question to the congregation.

He asked, "What do you have to do for the enemy to win?"

He then paused and looked down to gather his sermon notes and secure his Bible. He waited patiently and let the question settle in our minds as if he expected someone to blurt out the answer. The silence in the church grew, but no one spoke. He waited a few more moments and then looked back at the congregation, who at this point were eagerly awaiting the answer.

He then said, "In order for the enemy to win, all you have to do is nothing! Absolutely nothing!"

If we do nothing, the enemy wins! His answer was simple and true in so many ways. The enemy—Satan— wins in whichever areas of our lives we refuse to move with God.

The fact that I have a purpose on this earth to fulfill makes taking care of my body a must. What great idea, book, invention, or accomplishment has God created and ordained to be done through you? How will it be done if you're always battling unnecessary sickness or if you leave before your time? How hard would it be for you to accomplish your goals? Who's going to look after your loved ones or train them up in the way they should go? Who's going to do what only you can do? Whether we know it or not, we all have a God-ordained purpose. The purpose of being healthy is not what society has taught us as being true for our lives; rather, it is about what God has called you to do for His glory. It is about being at such a state of health that we can carry out His calling for our lives to our best abilities.

Even though physical fitness is not more important than spiritual fitness, it is important! We know our God is a God of order and that anything not in order is in chaos, and in that will He not abide. When we get in order we can receive the fullness of what He has for us. This fact is true in all the areas of our lives. When we don't position ourselves, we limit what God wants to do in and through us in that area. Our physical bodies should be viewed in the same light.

Our purpose is to advance the kingdom of God in the earth through the respective areas we are called to. We are to be fruitful and multiply with what He has given us to establish His kingdom. Whether you are a preacher, lawyer, cook, hairstylist, doctor, plumber, or athlete, those things and the like require a certain level of physical health. In every sphere of society, we are commissioned to take dominion and establish His government. For this reason our health is of great importance!

Five

IT'S NOT ABOUT YOU

A very important revelation is received when we understand that we have a purpose. It gives more understanding of why we are here and why our flesh has to die. It explains why God is always working on us—constantly changing, humbling us, and cleansing us of all selfish and unrighteous works.

When we understand we were created for a purpose, we understand that our lives and health are not about us. Our very lives are about someone else. It's about the glory of our Savior, our Redeemer, our king, being revealed through us. It's about His kingdom being established on earth as it is in heaven (Matthew 6:10). It's about us using our gifts to be a light that draws people everywhere to the knowledge of Jesus and His saving grace.

There are souls attached to us that will not reach their potential or slay their giants until we do. Someone's watching us, depending on us to lead the way. Someone needs our time, our prayers, our teaching, and our love. We have both good and bad examples of ones before us who have paved the paths we've either benefited or suffered from. What will you leave for those after you? What example will you give them to follow?

When I was younger and didn't know anything about purpose—or that I even had one—my only goal was to be a professional basketball player, make lots of money, get married, and give back to my family and a few charitable organizations. When the Lord called me and began to reveal my purpose, I realized how short-sighted and selfish I'd been. My first vision within myself was just about me, myself, and mine. God's vision will stretch you mentally, physically, and spiritually. You will work it, but you will not be able to accomplish it without the help of the Lord, nor will you be able to take the credit. It extends far beyond just you and your family, touching many.

> For God so loved the world, that he gave His only begotten Son, that whosoever believeth in Him should not perish, but have everlasting life. For God sent not His Son into the world to condemn the world: but that the world through Him might be saved. (John 3:16–17 KJV)

We all have an assignment from God to minister the gospel to others through the gifts and opportunities set before us, but what can we do if we don't take care of ourselves? The church is not the building where we have our worship services! *We* are the church, the temple of the spirit of God, and our calling, purpose, and commission extend far beyond where we've settled. "And He said unto them, Go ye into all the world, and preach the gospel to every creature" (Mark 16:15 KJV). The keyword in that scripture is *go*.

> The Lord is not slack concerning His promise, as some men count slackness; but is long-suffering to us-ward, not willing that any should perish, but that all should come to repentance. (2 Peter 3:9 KJV)

God wants all to be saved and needs vessels of purpose so that all humans might come to repentance, knowing that there is a God who gives life and life in abundance because they see His glory shining through us and His works being manifested.

If I told you that God would be coming to live in your home and use it as a base of operations from which He would establish His kingdom, what preparations or changes would you make to allow Him to feel comfortable and operate as He wills? What would you remove from your house? What would you clean up? What would you allow or not allow in your house? When we accept Jesus as our Lord and Savior, His spirit comes to live in us, not only to do a work in us but also through us (1 Corinthians 6:19–20).

Close your eyes and take some time to meditate on the scripture and questions that were just posed to you. Our God is a God of order, so for us to receive from Him or for Him to do a work through us, we have to be in the right position. We must be in order. Just like the question of what you would change if Jesus was coming to live at your home, the same changes you'd make for Him apply to our bodies! What are we hindering being done in the earth because we don't glorify God in our bodies?

Everything we do affects someone else, whether we know it or not. In order to be effective at anything you must take care of what you have been given to effect change. No matter our mission or goal—whether to be a congressman, a business owner, or just a good parent—we have to be physically fit. There is not a meaningful purpose on this earth that doesn't require this, and the more fit you are the more productivity and effectiveness you can potentially have in your life. Being physically fit gives us a larger capacity for service and potentially more effectiveness. When we are fit the things we must do will not be so physically taxing on our bodies but if we are slack in our health, we will have to exert more energy. "If the ax is dull and one does not sharpen the edge, Then he must use more strength; But wisdom brings success" (Ecclesiastes 10:10 NKJV).

We know that are bodies are the temple of the spirit of God who lives inside us. We are not our own, and as He is, so are we—servants! "Even as the Son of man came not to be ministered unto, but to minister, and to give His life a ransom for many" (Matthew 20:28 KJV).

How can we evangelize the sinner if we are unable to go to where they are? How can we operate in healing if our bodies are in chaos? How can we preach about a life of abundance when we are in bondage? Our health is one of the great examples to the lost that not only is Jesus our Savior, but our healer, who will sustain you if you trust him.

Our lives are to be a testimony to others about the goodness of God. We can't represent well what we don't live. It's time for us to get over ourselves. It's not about us! When we get that deep in our hearts that we are to effect change in the earth for the kingdom of God then can we look past our hurts and disappointments to fight for what God has given us access to through and by the power of the name that is above every name—*Jesus.*

Six

MIND OVER MATTER

Mind over matter is something my older cousin Tina said to me before I left for basic training in the US Army. I didn't have a full understanding of it at the time, but it would become clearer as I went along. If I could conquer what was in front of me in my mind, then I could conquer it in life. That statement is something that I still think about today and is just as true now as it was back then.

We all have obstacles and challenges in our lives that we must face, but we will never conquer them until we are able to put our minds—our faith—over matter. It is not until we are convinced of certain beliefs in our minds that we are able to conquer what we are facing.

When dealing with this issue, we must understand that convincing beliefs always determine our outward actions, whether they are healthy, positive beliefs or negative ones. Some of our problems lie in the fact that we don't know the truth, and others fear having negative results. This leaves one main area to cover for the battle of the mind: Do you believe God?

For us to win the battle of the mind we must first obtain truth. Truth is described in the *Merriam-Webster Dictionary* as the body of real things, events, and facts. It is the state of being the case and is sincerity in action, character, and utterance. The truth is something that is real or true. It is the real state of things or the body of real things. In the word of God, Jesus declares of Himself that, "I am the way the truth and the life" (John 14:6 KJV).

In the beginning was the Word, and Word was with God, and the word was God, The same was in the beginning with God. All things were made by Him; without Him was not anything made that was made. In Him was life; and the life was the light of men. And the light shineth in darkness; and the darkness comprehended it not. (John 1:1–5 KJV)

And the Word was made flesh, and dwelt among us and we beheld His glory, the glory as of the only begotten of the Father, full of grace and truth. (John 1:14 KJV)

God is truth, and we access that truth through Jesus Christ (John 1:17). The world denies daily the truth it has been searching for, and because of this, it will never have life until it repents and recognizes that God is the truth and Jesus is the door.

If we can accept that God is the absolute and above Him is no other authority and by no one else was creation framed or set. If we can accept that as the truth, then we can trust what He says. John describes God as the word and the Son of God (Jesus) as the living word. We can trust His word based on who He is, God!

All scripture is given by inspiration of God, and is profitable for doctrine, for reproof, for correction, for instruction in righteousness: That the man of God may be perfect, thoroughly furnished unto all good works. (2 Timothy 3:16-17 KJV)

On this battlefield it is important for us to renew our minds in the word and speak to our challenges and obstacles in faith, knowing that God's word is true and will work for us if we believe. There are many things we have accepted in our minds as the truth when it comes to our health, many of which have come from people we've trusted—either because we're related to them or because they're experts in their field. Therefore, we need the truth—the word of God—to distinguish between what is and isn't true.

What should be most natural to us is being covered up by deceptions and lies that manifest themselves before our eyes, leaving us believing that what we see is a set reality. The truth is that God has so much greater for us if we would just seek His kingdom first. You will not truly win the battle of the mind nor defend it successfully without the word of God to combat every lie of the enemy.

> For the word of God is quick, and powerful, and sharper that any two edged sword, piercing even to the dividing asunder of soul and spirit, and of the joints and marrow, and is a discerner of the thoughts and intents of the heart. (Hebrews 4:12 KJV)

The way of the world teaches us that sickness and untimely deaths are just to be expected and that you're lucky if you don't experience them. AIDS, cancer, high blood pressure, heart attacks, and the like are no more of the kingdom of God than is an innocent child being gunned down in a drive-by shooting. Everything we do, whether it's something or nothing, affects not only us but also those around us and those who come after us. In this is the importance of applying the truth of kingdom principles to our life that God has set in place for our health and wellbeing.

In the battle of the mind we must have faith. *Merriam-Webster Dictionary* describes faith as a belief and trust in and loyalty to God and a firm belief in something for which there is no proof. As mentioned earlier, we must not only seek the truth, but we must have faith in the holy character of God and believe that what he says is the absolute truth—even if our situation says otherwise.

"God is not a man that He should lie; neither the son of man that He should repent" (Numbers 23:19 NKJV).

"Now Faith is the substance of things hoped for, the evidence of things not seen" (Hebrews 11:1 NKJV).

It is the assurance of conviction that causes one to have a confident attitude toward God, believing that through Christ Jesus all things are possible. It's believing that God wants what's best for you, and that He's working things out for your benefit, even though you may not be able to see or feel it. God moves off of the faith that one shows in Him and His ability to meet every need. Without it, it is impossible to please Him (Hebrew 11:6).

When Satan attacks our lives, he does it to shake us and change the way we think so that we will begin to operate from a place off insecurity, doubt, fear, and defeat. Why? Because our body cannot lead; it can only follow! That leaves the responsibility of leadership ultimately to our flesh (sin nature), emotions, experiences, outside influence, and so on, void of God. We connect to God through His spirit in our heart (mind).

We connect to the world through our flesh. The building up of our spirit through a relationship with the Lord and by the renewing and washing of our minds in the water of His word will give victory in the battle of the mind. When we are not connected, Satan wins the battle, and ultimately our flesh will assume the role of leadership. That's exactly where he wants us and where God doesn't. At this state everything the enemy throws at us has impact, whereas in close relationship with the Lord we can rise above it.

Our emotions, flesh, and self-will left alone are like a fair-weather friend who is only happy when things are perfect and everything is going their way, but as soon as they don't get what they want they become moody and unstable. In that state you can't sustain or advance. After you make up your mind to go walking after work, this state will cause you to put it off for another day. That day becomes a week, then a month, and the next thing you know you have gone months with minimal effort toward your health. You begin to ride a roller coaster of emotional highs and lows packed with excuses.

Successfully winning the battle of the mind is of grave importance to every area of our lives—especially our health—because we are called to advance. Satan does not fear an immobile body, but a mobile one. this means he doesn't care about how powerful we are if we can't or are unwilling to go. We can't advance with unfit temples, and we will not stick to living healthy lifestyles with weak minds. What we are called to do for Christ requires spiritual, mental, and physical dedication. Together they are more beneficial to the advancement of the kingdom of God than they are separate. Our minds can work for us or against us. We will not win the battle of the mind until we are willing to repent, submit to God, and take on the mind of Christ.

We must renew our minds in prayer and in the word of God. This will change the way we think. The way we think will begin to change the way we talk. The way we talk will begin to cause us to will our bodies into action. I can't state how important this is, because one of the biggest hindrances to most people making healthy lifestyle choices and sticking with it is psychological barriers. Use the word of God, take it to battle and challenge what you have been previously taught by the world and life experiences as the truth.

I once heard a wise man say, "The mind is the most important asset to us, because if we take care of our mind, we can take care of everything else." Without a sound mind, we will always be subject to struggling and giving up on our goals. There are going to be some challenging days in the process to become healthy, but by having a strong mind in Christ you will be able to overcome.

On this journey to great health, resolve in yourself to depend on God for strength and wisdom. Trust in His word and follow His instruction. Meditate on His word, and renew your mind in it daily. Let it take you beyond your past failures and limits and past your insecurities, fears, and others' opinions to a place of faith in God that will give you the confidence to reach your goals. Stay consistent in the word and in prayer daily.

Avoid spending more time than you have to in negative atmospheres, whether that means not hanging out with certain people or going certain places or by not opening yourself up to certain music and television shows that counter your efforts to be positive. Instead spend your time doing things that will build positive changes in the mind. With unwavering faith in the mind, we can move mountains (Matthew 17:20). You can stand up to your circumstances and declare in faith that you are more than a conqueror through Him that loved us! (Romans 8:37).

Seven

EXERCISE YOUR GRACE

And God is able to make all grace abound toward you; that ye, always
having all sufficiency in all things, may abound to every good work.
—2 Corinthians 9:8 (KJV)

In this text, the apostle Paul is talking to the Corinthian church in
reference to the grace God has made available to them for good works.
After we've received Christ Jesus as our lord and savior, we are granted
grace. One of the functions of that grace is the God-given ability to
operate in ways and places we couldn't before. Grace is unmerited favor,
divine favor, or elegance of movement. Through Christ Jesus we have
favor that we did nothing to deserve. It's favor from the most-high God!
It's the ability to move in the true beauty of motion. Grace is what we
need to live a healthy life full of purpose.

For a body to perform any type of action, there must be a foundation
of muscle present. A muscle is a fixed bunch of fibers in the body, which
produce movement by contracting and dilating. We as living, functioning
beings use muscles to make various movements, like walking, jumping,
and throwing. Muscles also help in performing activities necessary for
growth and for maintaining a strong, healthy body. We have jaw muscles
that help us to chew food. We have muscles that move food through the
stomach and intestines to aid in digestion. We have muscles in the chest
to make breathing possible. The heart is a muscle that causes blood via
blood vessels to circulate throughout the body.

There are three types of muscle: skeletal, smooth, and cardiac. Skeletal muscles, also known as voluntary muscles, help to provide stability to the skeletal system. They help to produce movement and to stop it. Smooth muscles, also known as involuntary muscle because they are not under the conscious control of the brain, are found in various parts of the body, like the walls of the stomach, blood vessels, bladder, and the intestines. They help with functions in the body, like helping substances such as food in the digestive tract move through the body by producing slow, steady contractions. Cardiac muscles make up the wall of the heart. When the cardiac muscle cells contract, blood is then pushed out of the heart and into the arteries, circulating throughout the body and bringing nourishment to all the cells. That withstanding, all the actions of the muscles are limited in degree of movement and growth until birth.

As a baby in your mother's womb you were limited in your ability to move, grow, and develop. You were subjected to whatever your mother suffered through or supplied. Life had begun, but you hadn't started living yet. You were limited by the containment in the womb. It was not until your birth took place that your muscles were truly able to develop and grow.

From a spiritual view, before salvation we are all the same as a baby in the womb. We're limited in our ability to develop and completely subject to the confines of our flesh. Our lives have begun, but we haven't started living yet. Just as we were in our mother's wombs, we walked in the flesh in the ways of this world, sensing there was something greater without having the ability to move there. It is not until we are born again that we have access to a spiritual muscle called grace. We cannot reach the fullness of development and growth until this occurs. This grace is available to us only through Christ Jesus.

Grace and muscle are similar in this. We did not earn either of them, and if either is sedentary, they won't produce. Being sedentary means having little to no activity or movement. Living a sedentary lifestyle causes one to be unable to properly handle the stresses and opposing forces one's body faces in everyday life. We create strength and capacity for more when we push against the opposing force and force our body to adapt. Without the proper exercise, we will be unable to properly deal with life's challenges, like the stresses that come along with being a parent or the demands of our jobs.

Let's face it, when life hits, it hits hard, and there is nothing we can do to prevent it; however, we can learn how to respond to it properly. We can learn to work both physical and spiritual muscles in order to create the capacity within us for what we are dealing with or want to accomplish. God's grace allows for us not to be stuck in mediocrity, but instead gives us access to a higher level of achievement in every area of our lives, fitness being no exception.

We've all had setbacks concerning our health, but the great thing about grace and muscle is that they both allow for you to get back up every time you fall. The more you get up the stronger you get! "For a just man falls seven times, and riseth up again" (Proverbs 24:16 KJV).

> For if by one man's offense death reigned by one; much more they which receive abundance of grace and of the gift of righteousness shall reign in life by one, Jesus Christ. (Romans 5:17 KJV)

Grace and muscle are present throughout every stage of our life to assist us in our calling. God has provided us with enough of both to accomplish what he has placed us here to do, but we have to work them to maximize their potential in our life. "My grace is sufficient for you, for my power is made perfect in weakness" (2 Corinthians 12:9 NIV).

When we purchase anything new, there will often be instructions somewhere in the packaged item to explain what the product is and what its purpose is. These instructions were given by the creator, inventor, or manufacturer to instruct one on the right uses of the item, proper maintenance, warranty, and information explaining who to call in case of any problems beyond the purchaser's control.

Our creator is God, and our instruction manual is the word of God. Our customer service is the Holy Spirit. Oh! Don't worry about the bill; Jesus already paid it. He's given us a warranty in grace that lasts for all eternity. Without grace we cannot achieve what we have the potential to. Grace takes us from potential to actual fulfillment of what we are trying to obtain—or even better, what he has ordained us to attain.

Consider the fact that as a believer you may experience more resistance toward your efforts to live a healthy lifestyle because you are a threat to Satan's kingdom. Therefore, work the grace God has given you, and watch that muscle grow!

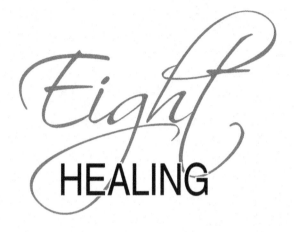

Eight
HEALING

Beloved, I wish above all things that thou mayest prosper
and be in health, even as thy soul prospereth.
—3 John 2 (KJV)

Before we can truly experience healing in our lives, we must understand where real healing comes from. We've been taught by our experiences and by society that healing rests in doctors' hands and in the medicines they prescribe. Pharmaceutical companies make billions off what we have been taught heals us. That couldn't be further from the truth!

Doctors play a very important role in our society, but it is not to heal us. Their function is of great importance, but that function is not healing. A doctor's primary job is to position us for our healing. Evidence of God's healing and sustaining power works in our bodies to some capacity every day, and we take it for granted.

Our bodies can heal from severe wounds, reform skin, and has the ability to recover from sickness. Not limited to the few listed, there are many examples of God's healing power at work in our lives. The reason this needs to be highlighted is because we put our faith for healing in the wrong places, people, and things. As stated before, the doctor's job is to position one for healing, not to produce it.

For example, there are plenty of medicines out there, but even if one is prescribed to you by a doctor, it is not guaranteed to be good for your body. I know I will catch a lot of heat, but I declare these things unto you! You would be hard pressed to find any drug that does not have some type of side effect, whether it is readily known or not.

Why would God give us anything that heals us in one area while causing problems in another? You will not find scripture to support healing with side effects. He is the God of more-abundant life! I posed this question earlier and I will present it again: If we were created by God, why are we using human-made solutions to fix a God-made body?

No medicine I've ever taken or have seen someone else take has ever healed them, but we still give the glory of healing to humans. At best, prescription drugs give us a temporary fix in order to allow our bodies to respond to an issue. They can kill bacteria, clean wounds, numb pain, or assist in an area, but the body still must respond for healing to take place.

If prescription drugs cured us, there would be little sickness and death among us. People who sell themselves the idea that these drugs do heal us find themselves with a plastic bag full of different prescription drugs and multiple side effects if they make it to old age. Their lives become more stressful—not only from the health issues, but from the financial hit they take to maintain it.

Most major businesses that market their products to us are not being led by the Spirit of God, but through humanity's limited knowledge. It does not matter a person's wisdom, knowledge, or good intentions, a carnal mind is in opposition to God and His will. It can't produce the perfect will of God.

We must take more of an interest in what is good for us and not leave a situation that needs godly wisdom to ones who do not seek or honor God. This does not mean you shouldn't take a drug prescribed by your doctor. Rather, you need to bring your faith up to a higher level where you believe we are healed by the stripes of Jesus and that He can show us how to better manage our health.

When I was in the eighth grade, I broke my ankle and tore a ligament while playing a pickup game of football. When I went to see the doctor about my injury, he took some x-rays and explained to me what he was going to do about it. He told me that they planned to fix the problem by surgically reconnecting the chipped bone and ligament to their original position. Then he explained they would leave it in a cast, and in the body's own timing, it would naturally heal on its own. The doctor did not heal me; he just put me in the best position for my body to heal itself.

I worked a job with my uncle replacing wooden floors in older homes. The working conditions were bad for my allergies, but I needed the work at the time—so I pressed on. Even though I wore a respiratory mask, I began to develop a severe allergic reaction that caused me to have a headache and consistent congestion over the following weeks, getting worse as time went on. I tried every sinus and allergy medicine I could buy without a prescription, but none of them worked. I prayed about it, but it did not clear up. It just seemed not to progress.

I finally went to see a doctor and was surprised by his response. After running some tests and asking a few questions, he concluded it was a sinus infection. The doctor seemed puzzled and commented that the infection seemed to have stopped in its tracks instead of getting any worse.

The doctor then explained to me that the body has natural defenses against things like sneezing, coughing, and runny noses. He explained that the medicines I had been taking that were designed to help me were instead drying out my system so that it couldn't respond properly. I believe even then the Lord was trying to get me to see humans' limited ability and understand that true healing was in Him. This doesn't mean that we won't ever use medicine or that we don't need doctors, but we need to put these things in proper perspective.

John the Baptist

"Repent for the kingdom of heaven has come near" (Matthew 3:2 NIV) was a statement made multiple times by one the most pivotal figures in biblical history, John the Baptist. John the Baptist was the forerunner to Jesus and had two primary messages to the people of that time.

The first message was to repent, and the second was that the Messiah, Jesus Christ, was coming and His kingdom with Him. John's assignment was not only to proclaim that the King was coming, but to prepare people's hearts and minds to receive Him. Doctors are the same in many way with regard to our health. Their assignment is to position us for our healing with information and practical application. They put our bodies in position to access healing, recover from an attack on our health, or to prevent damages to our current state of health.

Illusions or Healing?

What if I told you that what we have been taught or have accepted as healing through medicine is not true? As I've stated before, our bodies have been divinely created to heal themselves. A disconnect occurred at the fall of man which caused separation from God. It has caused us to experience difficulties God never intended concerning our health. Medicine has the ability to aid the body in the healing process, clean infected areas, suppress pain, or fight off things foreign to the body, but at the end of the day, when all is said and done, your body has to respond.

This puts the ball back in our court and supports what doctors have been fussing at us about for years—taking responsibility for our own health. What you do or don't do matters. We can take our vehicles to get fixed by a mechanic when we have problems beyond our expertise, but we at least need to know how to change a tire or recognize when something is wrong. It's our responsibility to know what type of fuel we need to put in our vehicle and when it is time to get the oil changed if we can't change it ourselves. Medicine may help if you're properly diagnosed but regardless your body must respond! If your body doesn't respond, then healing is not manifested.

Where Does Healing Start?

Our healing is brought about by first repenting and getting reconnected to the life source we've been disconnected from since the fall of man. This is made readily available through Christ Jesus by whose wounds we were healed (Isaiah 53:5, 1 Peter 2:24). Jesus has bridged the gap between us and God. It is not the Lord's will that we have cancer, AIDS, heart attacks, high blood pressure, or sexually transmitted diseases. It is not His will that we suffer needlessly.

If we were meant to suffer, why would God send His only son to give us abundant life (John 10:10)? Why did Jesus go about healing people of their infirmities and teaching His disciples to do the same in His name (Matthew 4:23, 10:1)? Why did Jesus declare that if we believe in Him, we shall do the works He has been doing and even greater works (John 14:12)? Healing is available to us—and it is for us—but in order to receive or maintain it there are some key principles we must apply. "Faith without works is dead" (James 2:20 NKJV).

Without faith it is impossible to please God (Hebrews 11:6), so we must first believe that the Lord can heal us. The word *works* stated to go along with faith does not mean that we make it happen, but rather it stands for an act of obedience toward an instruction symbolizing our faith that sets the atmosphere for or facilitates what God is getting ready to do.

The supernatural is almost always manifested in the application of a practical instruction that God gives. For example, God spoke to Noah and instructed him to build an ark. God was going to send a great rain to the earth that would cause a flood unlike anything that had ever been known to man. It would destroy both humans and beasts because of the wickedness of humans on the earth at that time.

Noah found grace with God so that he and his family, along with two of each creature, could be preserved. God gave Noah complete instructions on how to build the ark and what to build it with. God speaking to Noah was supernatural, but there was nothing supernatural about building an ark.

Noah practically applied God's instructions to him by faith, believing what he was told even though, at that point, humans had never experienced rain or a flood. Noah set an atmosphere through obedience to God's word, and because of it we are here today. His belief in God's word caused him to act, and humanity was preserved because of it.

I was in a church service one morning during which God healed everyone who came down to the altar. As each person came up, I heard in the Spirit, "You're healed; now get out of the way!" I meditated on that often after I heard it until God explained to me what He'd meant. He was saying that I was healed and now needed to stop living in a manner that could lead me back into the bondage from which I'd just been delivered. A good example of this is someone who carries a substantial amount of weight and develop a knee problem because of it. They go to be prayed for by the pastor and the elders of the church and receive their healing, but they never dealt with the *cause* of the knee problem—only the symptom. They are okay for a while, but weeks later the pain starts back and causes the person to become bitter and frustrated and may even start to lose faith.

It wasn't that God didn't heal that person. It was not that healing was not available. It was the fact that he or she lived the same way as before the healing. The excessive weight that caused the knee problem in the first place was never properly addressed, so it brought about the same problems as before. In order to truly walk in the healing God has for our lives we must repent (change our minds), trust God, and obey His instruction.

Many people think their circumstances will automatically change without obeying God's instructions in that area. It is possible to believe in God for something and nothing happens. Why? It wasn't because He did not make it available to us, but rather, we didn't follow the instructions given to facilitate what He wanted to do in our lives. If it is in His will to do what we are asking for, the next question should be: Am I in His will? Am I in position to receive what I'm believing for?

We must trust God to be who He says He is and trust that He is willing and more than able to meet our needs. We must listen for and obey His practical instruction for us. Then we must act in obedience to His instruction. When we do those things, we're able to grab hold of what He has already released to us. We must remember that it is not our actions that cause the healing to manifest but our faith in the healing power of Jesus that causes us to act on whatever He has instructed us to do.

We must apply God's principles concerning health to our lives. The results of the kingdom of God cannot be produced through any area in which we refuse to submit to Him. I don't care how great of an athlete you are, how slim you are, or how much muscle you possess. If you do not apply His principles concerning health to your life, it will catch up with you!

There have been a number of body builders over the years who had completely ripped, muscled bodies and died from kidney failure. Ex-football players in their forties and fifties die suddenly of heart attacks after being physically active for most of their lives. There have been high school athletes who have mysteriously dropped dead in the middle of games. Sickness and death do not respect people, but they both must bow at the name of Jesus. Know who your healer is, and apply His principles to your life.

> If thou will diligently hearken unto the voice of the Lord thy God, and wilt do that which is right in His sight, and wilt give ear to His commandments, and keep all His statutes, I will put none of these diseases upon thee, which I have brought upon the Egyptians: for I am the Lord that healeth thee. (Exodus 15:26 KJV)

> "Let us return to our healer, who heals all our diseases" (Psalm 103:1–3 NIV).

> "For there is healing in His wings" (Malachi 4:2 KJV).

Nine

CREATOR'S CHOICE

When it comes to the question of what we should eat, one should consider eating to live and not living to eat. Nothing that God has created for us to eat causes negative effects in our body in and of itself. It is only when one eats in error or in a gluttonous manner does this change. The bible teaches us that this type of lifestyle will leave one poor and clothed with rags "Do not join those who drink too much wine or gorge themselves on meat, for drunkards and gluttons become poor, and drowsiness clothes them in rags" (Proverbs 23:20–21 NIV).

Yes, food is delicious, and we are to enjoy it but should always keep proper perspective. We should first view food as fuel. Meaning you eat in order to fuel your body's functions. This says you will put the right things in your system in order for it to perform the way God intended. Very rarely does the average person ask what they should eat for health, but it is just as important as anything else. As soon as our bodies tell us it's hungry, more times than not our minds immediately gravitate toward what we desire over of what is good for us. Our bodies are asking for fuel, but we have been conditioned to register hunger from a carnal perspective and not from a place of what we need.

We also have the effects of eating highly processed foods that have addictive qualities. The fast food industry is making a killing off of our misconception, leaving our bodies depleted and wanting more. We are depleted because what we have consumed rarely meets the needs of the body. We are left wanting because our bodies never got what they were asking for in the first place, which was nourishment. So we leave our bodies unequipped to fight. Our bodies were created to perform with the use of foods created by God, unaltered by humans.

Genesis 1:29 and 2:15–3:24 tell the account of the fall of man. After placing Adam in the garden of Eden, God instructed him about what to eat. The only thing he was not allowed to eat from in the garden was the fruit from the tree of the knowledge of good and evil. In disobedience to God Adam and his wife, Eve, ate fruit from the tree. The consequence was the fall of humanity.

> "By one man's offense death reigned by one" (Romans 5:17 KJV).

> "For one man's disobedience many were made sinners" (Romans 5:19 KJV).

That's powerful! That one action of disobedience would affect every generation after it in a negative way. The magnitude of this action is of great importance for us to understand because any disregard of God's set principles is a form of rebellion. When we rebel against God or His principles, it causes separation from Him and chaos—specifically in the area in which we rebelled.

In the space of separation from God, sickness and untimely death have room to come into our lives. If we take God and His principles out of our finances we allow for sickness and death to come in the form of debt. If we rebel against God by fornicating, we allow sickness and death in the form of sexually transmitted diseases. If we take God out of our marriages, we allow sickness and death in the form of divorce, adultery, dysfunction, and the like. We can have a life of great health on this earth until our appointed time if we apply God's principles; grace by Jesus Christ has granted us access (Romans 5:17).

What's Best for Us (the Essentials)

Contrary to popular belief, God never intended for man or animals to be eaters of meat.

> And God said, "Behold, I have given you every herb bearing seed, which is upon the face of all the earth, and every tree, in the which is the fruit of a tree yielding seed; to you it shall be for meat. And to every beast of the earth, and to every fowl of the air, and to everything that creepeth upon the earth, wherein there is life, I have given every green herb for meat: and it was so." (Genesis 1:29–30 KJV)

The meaning of the word *meat* in the early seventeenth century when the King James Version of the bible was translated as *food*. The actual eating of meat from animals was prohibited until after the great flood. God specifically made certain foods to fuel our bodies. This confirms biblically that a plant-based diet of fruits, vegetables, nuts, and grains should be the foundation of our everyday diet.

Our bodies need naturally grown produce above any other food source. We were built to thrive on them. Plant-based foods are loaded with all the vitamins, nutrients, and minerals our bodies need to function properly without being high in calories. They also contain natural enzymes that allow our bodies to readily absorb what is in them.

Yes, humans were created with the ability to eat and survive on food from both plants and animals. However, we were created to consume and anatomically respond to plant-based diets. If possible, choose organic over any other form of produce. You should be able to find good choices in healthy grocery stores. Also support your local farmers and farmers markets. We need to put a greater demand on our government to produce more organically grown produce.

One of the biggest questions I hear pertaining to a plant based diet, especially when talking about fitness, is where you can get protein if you don't eat meat. Strangely that and just being used to eating meat seem to be the only objections. You can get protein in your diet from boiled soybeans, lentils, large white beans, cranberry beans, split peas, pinto beans, kidney beans, black beans, navy beans, lima beans, lentil, quinoa, tempeh, chickpea, tofu, chia seed, edamame, industrial hemp, soy milk, seitan, nut, almond, spinach, broccoli, peanuts, legumes, wild rice, sprouted bread, and more. It has been heavily marketed that animal protein and its byproducts are the only major sources of protein. That's funny because most animals we humans eat for protein eat a plant-based diet themselves.

Water

The most important source of nutrition for the body is water. Vital to almost every function of the body, water makes up two-thirds of a person's body weight. Our bodies can't go more than three to five days without it, whereas a body can go nearly a month without food. A necessary part of bodily functions, water flushes waste products, revitalizes the body, lubricates the joints, prevents dehydration, and is good for the skin. Water helps slow the aging process and prevents problems in the kidneys by keeping them flushed out. Water is also necessary to regulate blood pressure in people with high cholesterol levels, diabetes, hiatal hernias, allergies, constipation, gastrointestinal matter, headaches, angina, hypertension, and obesity.

Water functions as a combination of compounds, transporter, reactant, and a principle of gaseous diffusion. Water also protects moving organs, provides body volume and form, thermoregulates body temperature, and is used in the balance of chemicals and as an ingredient in cellular metabolism. It is the most functional nutrient in our body and is also a noncaloric beverage. The growls in our stomach we associate with hunger are often indicators of thirst. We usually fail to give our bodies the needed water and wrongly assume we need more food. A very large portion of our population, walk around dehydrated or are very close to it and don't realize it.

Regardless of your level of activity, your body can only go so far without water, so make it the most frequent beverage in your diet. It is literally a liquid life source and very significant to our survival. So much so that Jesus uses it as a reference to life in Him and a symbol of His spirit. "But whoever drinks the water I give them will never thirst. Indeed, the water I give them will become in them a spring of water welling up to eternal life" (John 4:14 NIV).

Consumption of Meat

After the great flood in Genesis, Noah and his sons were given permission from God to eat meat. After Moses led the children of Israel out of Egypt, God gave him a list of the animals to be considered clean or unclean for consumption, for they were to be set apart from other nations. For a list of these meats, see Leviticus 11 and Deuteronomy 14. Even though there are plenty of meats we can eat that have some nutritional value, they should be limited in their consumption and portion size. We are commanded in the word of God not to be among those who are riotous eaters of meat (Proverbs 23:20).

Just like everything God does, He does it purposefully and without mistakes. So if God commanded His people to do something, it was not just to say it. There are both spiritual and natural implications behind everything God does. This is not to bring people back under the law, because we are under grace. With that said, there are always reasons God does things, and for that reason it is worth looking into the matter.

It would be wise for us to stick to the list of clean and unclean meats listed in the word of God. Many people use the vision of Peter in Acts 10, to validate the consumption of all meat, but that was a reference to salvation now being available to all men. In the beginning of Acts 10:1–28, we read about a devout centurion named Cornelius whose lifestyle of generosity and prayers came up as a memorial to the Lord. He was commanded by an angel of the Lord to send for Peter who would instruct him on what he needed to do.

In the same text Peter is recorded having a vision concerning meats that were considered unclean for him as a Jew to eat. Peter responded according to the law when God told him to kill and eat. The bible states that while Peter was praying he fell into a trance and had a vision where all manner of four-footed beasts and creeping things and fowls of the air were let down to him from an opened heaven in a vessel that looked like a sheet knit at the four corners.

He hears a voice say to him, "Rise, Peter. Kill and eat."

Peter responds by saying, "Not so, Lord, for I've never eaten anything that is common or unclean."

This was spoken to Peter three times before he was commanded not to call what God has cleansed common. This is where I've seen most people stop and set up camp concerning this text, but if you read all the way up to the twenty-eighth verse, Peter explains that God showed him in the dream that he shouldn't call any *human*—not animal—common or unclean. Peter was a Jew, and he explains in verse 28 that it was unlawful for a Jew to keep company with or to come unto one of another nation. Cornelius was a gentile, and before him Peter had never dealt with gentiles. God was telling Peter that He had made salvation available to all humans. This should not be used as a reference toward what meats we can consume.

Once again, this is not to bring anyone back under the law, so don't come under condemnation. I just want you to simply understand that God does everything for a reason, and it just so happens that eating by God's standard is better for your health. It has been proven that the consumption of meat—especially when it's highly processed meat—can lead to many of the diseases many in our society suffer from, like high blood pressure, obesity, and can even cancer. No, you are not going to hell for eating meat, but you can open a door for sickness and even untimely death the further away from God's plan you eat. When pondering the pros and cons of eating certain foods it is important to remember that even though you might have the power to choose, you must consider whether it is of any benefit to your health.

> "All things are lawful unto me, but all things are not expedient: all things are lawful for me, but I will not be brought under the power of any" (1 Corinthians 6:12 KJV).

Most of our unhealthy fats come from a meat-heavy diet. Meat from wild game will usually be the healthiest source of meat barring potential pollution from its environment. Wild game fat content usually run under 10 percent, whereas fat from domesticated animals can be three times higher—or more. It would be wise to stay clear of highly processed meat.

When it comes to nutrition, this is the foundation.

I know what you're thinking—*this can't be all there is to it?* But fundamentally, it is. The proper consumption of what I just explained to you, along with daily exercise, is what will help you get to your goals. Outside of any unknown complication that may be unique to a particular person, it's that simple. We should always measure what man has said is OK for us to consume against what the word of God says. God is the Creator, and we are not! God is always right, without fail; we are not. A lot of the things that make living a healthy lifestyle difficult disappear when we submit to God's plan.

Processed (Altered) Foods

Every form of food comes from some type of natural source, whether it is plant or animal based. If it doesn't, I don't recommend you eat it. Everything we consume from potato chips to honey buns should come from some type of natural food source. At this point the question we should ask is: If all the ingredients in the food are natural, what type of process did this food source go through to get to what is being presented in front of me now? What process was taken to make it taste like it does? What did humans alter; what did they add to this food that caused it to be what it is?

This goes back to what was said about false prophets. They will take a truth and twist it just enough for it to appear to be truth, even though it's not. It appears to be good, but just like Adam and Eve in the garden, when we partake of it, sickness and death come into our lives. Now we must count calories when in times past that was not an issue.

Now we must go on specialized diets and take different supplements and medicines in an attempt to attain good health.

Ask yourself this question: Why would God create something to eat that would make me sick? He wouldn't! This only happens when humans operate in their own wisdom. Any compromise or misuse of what God has created will eventually have the consequences of anything void of Him. It will breed sickness and death in some shape, form, or fashion. When dealing with processed foods we must consider what has been altered by humans in that food from the beginning.

A lot of food manufacturers' bottom lines are about profit and not sound doctrine. Now don't get me wrong, when you're in business you must make money, or you won't last long. But making money should not be done at the expense of people's health. Corners are cut for the sake of taste, low pricing, and longer shelf lives. All types of actors, athletes, and so on are paid millions of dollars to star in commercials promoting these products instead of the manufacturers putting efforts into the quality of their food.

I have news for you, friends; there is no such thing as a 99.9 percent truth. It's either the truth or a lie. It is either a true presentation, or it's not. Compromise not only affects the food, but also how the food affects us. Will this yield the same benefits to me as it would in its most natural state, or will the changes made to it put my body in a vulnerable position? Foods prepared in ways that do not compromise their nutritional values will always be more beneficial to you.

Quality of food is worth more than having an abundance of it. We must always consider the process and preparation of the food we eat. With the use of money for advertising, companies entice us with appealing offers, depicting scenes of great times with family and friends to play on our emotional and fleshly desires. As mentioned earlier, they use professional athletes and entertainers to influence their target markets. One fast food chain was notorious for using Olympic athletes in its commercials, but if you'd looked at the athletes' actual training diets, I doubt you'd have seen fast foods or any other highly processed foods on it.

The effects that highly processed foods have on the body can cause you to battle sickness and unnecessary weight gain more often. This can be immediate or accumulated over a period of time. Highly processed foods can have a negative effect on the natural processes of the body, like your metabolism, thus hindering your body from doing what it is supposed to with the food you ingest.

I believe there will soon be more and more studies that link diseases and the like to the processed foods we eat. To be honest, the health of our society is in just as much of a need of change than many countries where people are without proper amounts of food. Our problem does not lie in whether we have enough, but whether we have enough of what was created for us? The food God created for us to eat caters to life, whereas human-altered food may not fall in line with that standard.

For those who are saddened by this information and want to know what can be done to replace these different foods, snacks, and desserts we love so much, have no fear. I have great news! The enemy cannot create. He can only copycat something that has already been created. As believers we know that what happens in the natural realm (what we can see) comes after something has happened in the spiritual realm (what we can't see). We also know that what God has for us does not produce negative side effects.

So if there is a negative presentation of something—let's just use the honey bun for instance—then there must be a positive version of the honey bun that's healthy for us to eat as well as delicious. The problem is—where is it? It's waiting for a kingdom-minded cook or nutritionist to tap into the spiritual realm and grab hold of it.

From the information I've already shared, we know that the majority of what we should consume as food should be natural and brought forth from the earth along with water. Biblically this qualifies as a complete diet. Even though God allows us to eat meat we should remember that it was not His original plan for us, so we should limit our consumption of it and adhere to the list of clean and unclean animals in Leviticus 11 and Deuteronomy 14. Highly processed foods are not recommended. When looking for places to eat out, mom-and-pop restaurants are more likely to serve fresh organic products. Even though you may get more for your buck, stay away from the buffet if you have self-control issues. Sometimes eliminating the power to choose is the best form of self-control.

If you're looking to lose some weight, first you must address your body's health. Weight gain, just like sickness, is a symptom of dysfunction in the body. When we eat right, we support how God intended our bodies to function. When our bodies are at a place of health, they will begin to work for us. When we operate according to God's principles, we will always see results!

Ten
IT TAKES BALANCE

On your journey to good health, it will take balance to achieve your desired goals. *Balance* as defined by the *Merriam-Webster Dictionary* as physical equilibrium. Without proper balance you will hinder your efforts. Lack of balance in a person's life—especially when dealing with health—is often overlooked and is rarely emphasized. This fact can either make or break you on your journey to good health. There is no healthy shortcut around this! The important elements you leave out or try to cheat on will not only make it hard on you, but will also have the potential to stop you.

There are elements to balance that are very important on your health journey. The first of these is a having a *sound spiritual life.* As a believer, if you take any step toward the purpose for which you were created, you can rest assured there will be spiritual opposition from the enemy. The car will break down, insecurities will pop up, people will start offering you food you know you don't need to eat, and the daily demands of life will seem to go into overdrive. It would be so easy to say that you don't have enough time or energy to get in shape. For this reason, you need strength beyond yourself to accomplish your goals. We need a helper!

> But you will receive power when the Holy Spirit comes
> on you; and you will be my witnesses in Jerusalem, and
> in all Judea and Samaria, and to the ends of the earth.
> (Acts 1:8 NIV)

One of the functions of the Holy Spirit is to give you power to do what you could not do in your own strength. God does not give us purposes that we can do in our own strength, nor does He create us to live void of Him. We need Him to live! True greatness is in God, and no great or noteworthy accomplishment is done without Him. He is the beginning of all knowledge and truth, and He will never leave you or forsake you on your journey. He is the answer to every problem. If you keep Him first, you will be able to make it. He is your source of strength when you are spiritually, physically, or mentally drained. "He will strengthen you with might by His spirit in the inner man" (Ephesians 3:16 KJV).

> I know what it is to be in need, and I know what it is to have plenty. I have learned the secret of being content in any and every situation, whether well fed or hungry, whether living in plenty or in want. I can do all this through him who gives me strength. (Philippians 4:12–13 NIV)

Learn to depend on God. We can do nothing without Him, and without Him, we are nothing. Be careful to desire Him and not just what He can do for you. Everything else will be taken care of if we delight ourselves in Him with a sincere heart. The Lord is our refuge, our very life source through Jesus, by whom the foundations of our lives should be built upon! Through relationship with Him, wage good warfare!

Secondly, we must have *proper nutrition.* Without the proper foods in our system we cannot expect to achieve the levels of fitness we desire. You might be thinking, *I have a relative who eats however they want and never seem to gain a pound.* Just because someone has a slim figure doesn't mean they are healthy. There are graveyards and hospitals full of individuals who appeared to be fit but struggled with their health. Because we are all unique, improper nutrition does not always have the same appearance, except for the fact it impacts our bodies in a negative way.

Improper nutrition often has a cumulative effect on our bodies that impacts us later down the line. God has created our bodies to process certain foods for fuel. It is to us as gas and oil are to a car. If we don't have it, we can't go! Our bodies will respond by underperforming and eventually failing. The practices that cause malnutrition are something that, if not addressed early, will be on to the next generation in consequence or in the form of bad habits. We have seen the signs already in the growing obesity rate in children. Proper nutrition replenishes the body and gives it fuel to go. Exercise without it can put your body through undue stress just like an engine being pushed while low on oil.

Exercise goes hand in hand with proper nutrition. It is very important to be active in both of those areas in order to get the best results. Stress can be measured in two ways: negative and positive. Negative stress is the type of stress that is of no benefit to us, like worrying. Negative stress can impact both our physical and mental health—like the stress we get from bad relationships or when we stress over being behind on our bills.

Positive stress is a type of stress you can benefit from. This can be created by positive challenges or the right view of negative ones. Parents, mentors, and coaches are examples of people who can push or motivate you to become better by providing an atmosphere of positive stress in your life. Exercise is a form of positive stress that, when done correctly, causes your body to respond in a positive manner according to the stress put on it. It can improve our health, energy, productivity, and appearance. It can slow the process of aging and early functional decline. Exercise can also help prevent and determine how well or how soon our bodies can recover from illness. Doctors often prescribe exercise to their patients to prepare their bodies for the stresses of an upcoming surgery and afterward to insure proper recovery.

As we get older, we normally began to slow down and participate in little or no exercise. We fall into the trap of self-preservation and stop moving. The exact opposite is needed! Proper exercise can increase vitality, even in the elderly. It has been scientifically proven that substantial muscle gain can be achieved in people who we perceive as over the hill. Exercises that include resistance have been proven to increase bone density. No, you might not be able to move like you used to, but you can be at a state of health in which you're able look and feel younger and also do more than the average person in your age range. If there is breath in your body, there is room for positive change.

Proper rest may be one of the most underrated elements to fitness. Our society teaches us to work long and hard hours to get where we want in life. Cram as much as you can in a short period of time, get little sleep, and if that doesn't work, get less. I believe in hard work, but that does not eliminate the need for rest. Sometimes we are required to make those types of sacrifices, but we must ask ourselves whether it's God's will for our lives or if we need to make some changes. Regardless of what anyone has told you, getting proper rest plays one of the biggest roles in you having a balanced and healthy life. At rest is when your body goes into the maintenance stage and begins to repair and replenish itself from the past days' work in preparation for the next. In this stage the combination of rest and nutrition play a big part in your body's ability to recover. Exercise also helps in this process by increasing your body's ability to rest and recover. It is important to get as much done as you can in life, but it is just as important to rest.

When we are well rested, we are more efficient and productive in our work. We make better decisions and reduce the chances of mistakes and accidents. When we are tired and trying to do too much, we end up drawing a lot of things out longer than need be. We become irritable and less productive. We also increase our chances of becoming sick due to a weaker immune system. We are more beneficial to our purposes when we are well rested. This means that we can't do everything.

I was wisely advised that sometimes you have to learn to say the anointed word *no*! This doesn't mean that I don't help others. It just means that I recognize I'm human and need adequate rest to function to my best ability. We must realize it's not just about whether God can use us, but rather how consistent and productive we can be when called upon. Eventually something worn down will break, and what could have been a lifetime of good works becomes just a work or two.

It is a requirement and our God-given responsibility to be good stewards of our bodies. We will always have those who need some type of help or something we feel needs to be done. I'm not encouraging not to help or to do whatever you have to do to reach your goals in life, but rather to take care of yourself while doing it.

> "And God blessed the seventh day, and sanctified it:
> because that in it he had rested from all his work which
> God created and made" (Genesis 2:3 KJV).

Proper rest is essential to a purpose-driven life, and we won't get as far as we think we can without it! God is self-sufficient and needs no rest. We, on the other hand, are God dependent, so we need times in prayer, fellowship with other believers, vacations with family, and other forms of rest and getting away from the normal flow of life to maintain a good balance. Those who spend a lot of their time pouring out need some time to get away and be poured into to prevent burnout.

Personal hygiene, which is often overlooked, is defined as the preservation of health. Bad hygiene can leave the body at a weak and vulnerable state. What we put in our bodies as well as on our bodies can affect our health. Food, medicine, and even lotions can affect us in a negative way if they consist of harmful ingredients that interfere with the normal functions of the body. Personal cleanliness aids in our bodies' defenses against communicable diseases, like the flu, and prevents the accumulation of bacteria. Bad hygiene can affect you socially and can also be a sign of depression or mental illness. Personal hygiene may seem like a small issue, but it has the ability to affect broad areas of our health.

Finally, we have *education.* Just as our bodies require exercise to maintain or improve upon our health, so do our minds. If we don't work our minds, just like anything else, it will not work for us. Mental challenges do for our minds what weights do for our bodies. Don't be afraid to challenge your mind with higher education or with exercises that make you think and focus. Read more, and set goals for yourself. Take some time to learn about how your body works.

No one should know more about your body than you. Don't back down from challenges that make you think critically. Your mind needs those challenges to help maintain where you are and to facilitate growth. It's not possible to *do* better until we *know* better. We must allow God to break down those barriers in our minds that we've allowed to be so firmly established. Expose your mind to the fullness of God. He's limitless in what He has to offer you.

Everything we do or don't do influences something or someone in our lives. Having a balance of a sound spiritual life, proper nutrition, rest, exercise, good hygiene practices, and education will enhance your life. The opposite can increase stress and instability in the body, hindering your ability to be productive in what God has called you to.

It will affect the way God can use you, because He will not violate His laws to pacify our laziness.

If we don't get in line with His order, we can't expect His kingdom to be manifested in our lives. Each of the six elements I've listed will affect what you can or can't do, and the sufficiency of each affects your overall production. I encourage you to live a life of balance. Your body will thank you for it, and others will benefit from it as you accomplish God's purpose for your life.

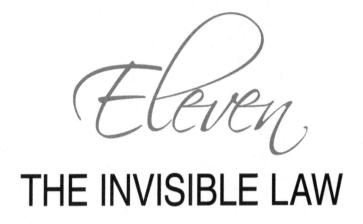

THE INVISIBLE LAW

Be not deceived; God is not mocked: for whatsoever a man
soweth, that shall he also reap. For he that soweth to his
flesh shall of the flesh reap corruption: but he that soweth
to the Spirit shall of the Spirit reap life everlasting"
—Galatians 6:7–8 (KJV)

There is an invisible law that holds true no matter what your personal beliefs are. That is the law of the seed—that whatever a man sows he shall reap. Whatever man puts his time and effort into or whatever he gives himself to, he will reap it. Sir Isaac Newton's third law of motion states that for every action, there is an equal and opposite reaction. With everything we do, there is a set stage for reaping, whether it is something positive or negative. No matter what, there will be a reaping or consequence from what is sown. So if one lives a life of perversion and corruption, they will reap a harvest of the same. If one sows the seed of an unhealthy lifestyle they will reap of it, but if one sows into the things of the Spirit they shall reap life.

When we look at the law of the seed from a purpose perspective and see the lives that God has called us to impact, we will understand our choices matter—even from an early age. They affect more than just us. There is no such thing as your choices not affecting others. Therefore, it is of great importance to sow good seed, because our lives are truly—at the core—not about us but about God and what He wants us to do to reconcile the lost back to Him.

So your physical health is not about your physique more than it is about whether you can produce. When people see your life, do they see the kingdom of God in full operation, or do they see someone who looks and operates exactly like them trying to win them to Christ?

Start sowing seeds of healthy living now. No matter how challenging it may seem, we must continue forward, even when we don't feel we are making much progress. We must be consistent in living a healthy lifestyle and while we are actively waiting, He will give the increase (1 Corinthians 3:6). Taking care of oneself is a good thing and is pleasing to God, so don't grow weary in it.

In steadfastness and dedication we will reap in due season (Galatians 6:9). If you are lacking strength call on God, His strength is made perfect in weakness (2 Corinthians 12:9). He will perfect, establish, strengthen, and settle you (1 Peter 5:10).

Sow good seeds in the form of positive habits and lifestyle choices, for surely you will reap a harvest!

FINAL THOUGHTS

There is so much we can learn about our health, and my prayer is that this book has been a tool to give you some revelatory insight on the topic. I pray you were able to grab something for your life. I've been applying these principles to my life and have already seen God move in a mighty way, and I look forward to seeing greater in my life and in yours.

God has a tremendous call on your life, and He is not a respecter of persons but rather can and will use anyone who is willing.

We have a purpose, but you can't fulfill it without taking better care of yourself. Ecclesiastes 10:10 teaches us that if our axe is dull and we don't sharpen the edge, more strength is needed, but if we apply wisdom to the situation that is sharpening the edge, it will bring success. Exercising our bodies and our minds are ways that we can sharpen our edge.

By giving our lives to Jesus Christ, who reconciles us to the father, we are mercifully given access to grace, forgiveness, healing, power, identity, and direction, through which we are to fulfill the assignment of establishing His kingdom throughout the earth. The journey to good health is not always easy, but it is necessary—not just for our sakes, but for the work of our callings in Christ Jesus. The world is dying all around us, headed for eternal damnation. What are you going to do about it?

As you think about the things you learned in this book and about the things you know must be changed, done away with, or altered in your life. As you set your heart on being greater in the areas of health and purpose in your life, I want you to meditate on the following scripture.

> Is not this the fast that I have chosen? To loose the bonds of wickedness, to undo the heavy burdens, and to let the oppressed go free, and that ye break every yoke? Is it not to deal thy bread to the hungry, and that thou bring the poor that are cast out to thy house? When thou seest the naked, that thou cover him; and that thou hide not thyself from thine own flesh? Then shall thy light break forth as the morning, and thine health shall spring forth speedily: and thy righteousness shall go before thee; the glory of the Lord shall be thy reward. Then shalt thou call, and the Lord shall answer; thou shalt cry, and he shall say, Here I am. If thou take away from the midst of thee the yoke, the putting forth of the finger, and speaking vanity; And if thou draw out thy soul to the hungry, and satisfy the afflicted soul; then shall thy light rise in obscurity, and thy darkness be as the noonday: And the Lord shall guide thee continually, and satisfy thy soul in drought, and make fat thy bones: and thou shalt be like a watered garden, and like a spring of water, whose waters fail not. And they that shall be of thee shall build the old waste places: thou shalt raise up the foundations of many generations; and thou shalt be called, The repairer of the breach, The restorer of paths to dwell in. (Isaiah 58:6–12 KJV)

May God bless you in all of your efforts to pursue Him! I pray that you attain all that He has for you in Jesus's name!

Printed in the United States
by Baker & Taylor Publisher Services